Ageing
A Milestone

**Important facts and
Personalised health care diary**

NEWBEE PUBLICATION

Copyright © 2020 Newbee Publication All rights reserved

This book should not be reproduced, stored, transmitted in any form or by any means without the publisher's written permission.

Disclaimer

This book has been written as a self-management guide for older adults and is not intended to replace medical professionals' advice in any way. To the extent possible, the author has made every effort to share updated information to date. The author accepts no liability for any loss, injury, or damage to any person due to the booklet's contents.

This Diary Belongs to

_____

If misplaced, please return to this address:

_____

_____

Or Contact: _____

Preamble

Ageing! Everyone perceives this word differently; some read as getting older, some as a ticket to freedom, some as anxiety and depression. As I know, Ageing is a milestone. A milestone that every single person will come across at later stages of life. This diary will help you on this journey of achieving an ageing milestone and inform you about the hitches of this journey so that you are fully prepared to enjoy this trip.

This diary contains essential information, and spaces are given to note down important information about yourself or past experiences related to your health.

You can keep this diary whenever you are going out on holidays or for an outing, in case of emergencies; the doctor can read your health concerns and guide you or treat you accordingly.

Everyone does not need to come across all the problems stated in this book. The writer aims to acquaint you with the process and empower you to be vigilant of issues and manage them effectively with a collaborative approach. Consider suggestions as a piece of advice from a well-wisher who is working in the community with older adults. There is no intention to scare you or deter you from seeking medical advice.

At the end of the book, a home-based exercise programme is given as a guideline, and you can customise it according to your needs.

List of Prescribed Medicines

Medicine	Time	Days

Medicine in case of emergency
_____
_____

Important Contact numbers

Names	Contact number	Remarks
ICE (in case of emergency)		
NOK (next to Kin)		
Doctor		
Ambulance		
Gas Leakage		
Pharmacy		

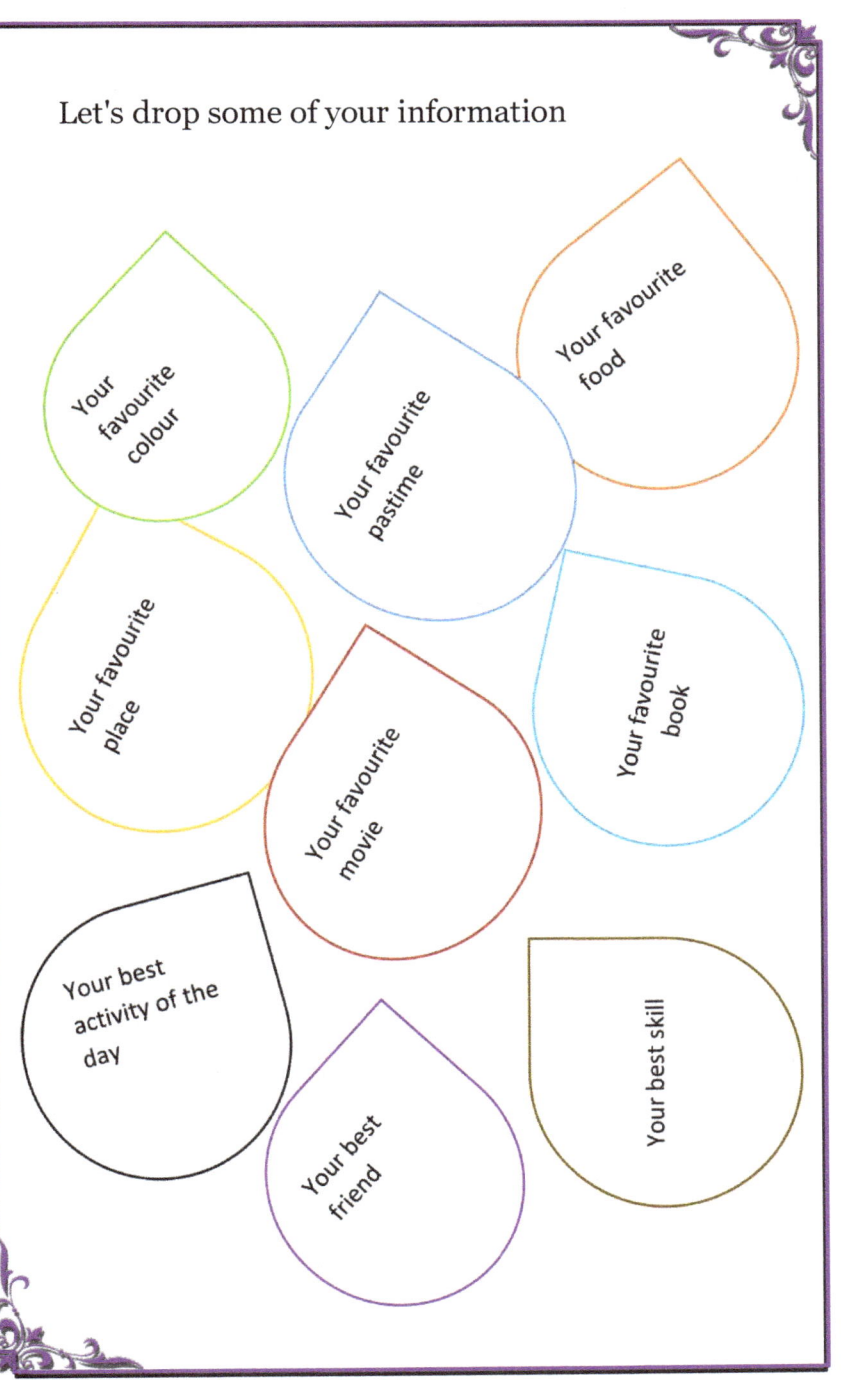

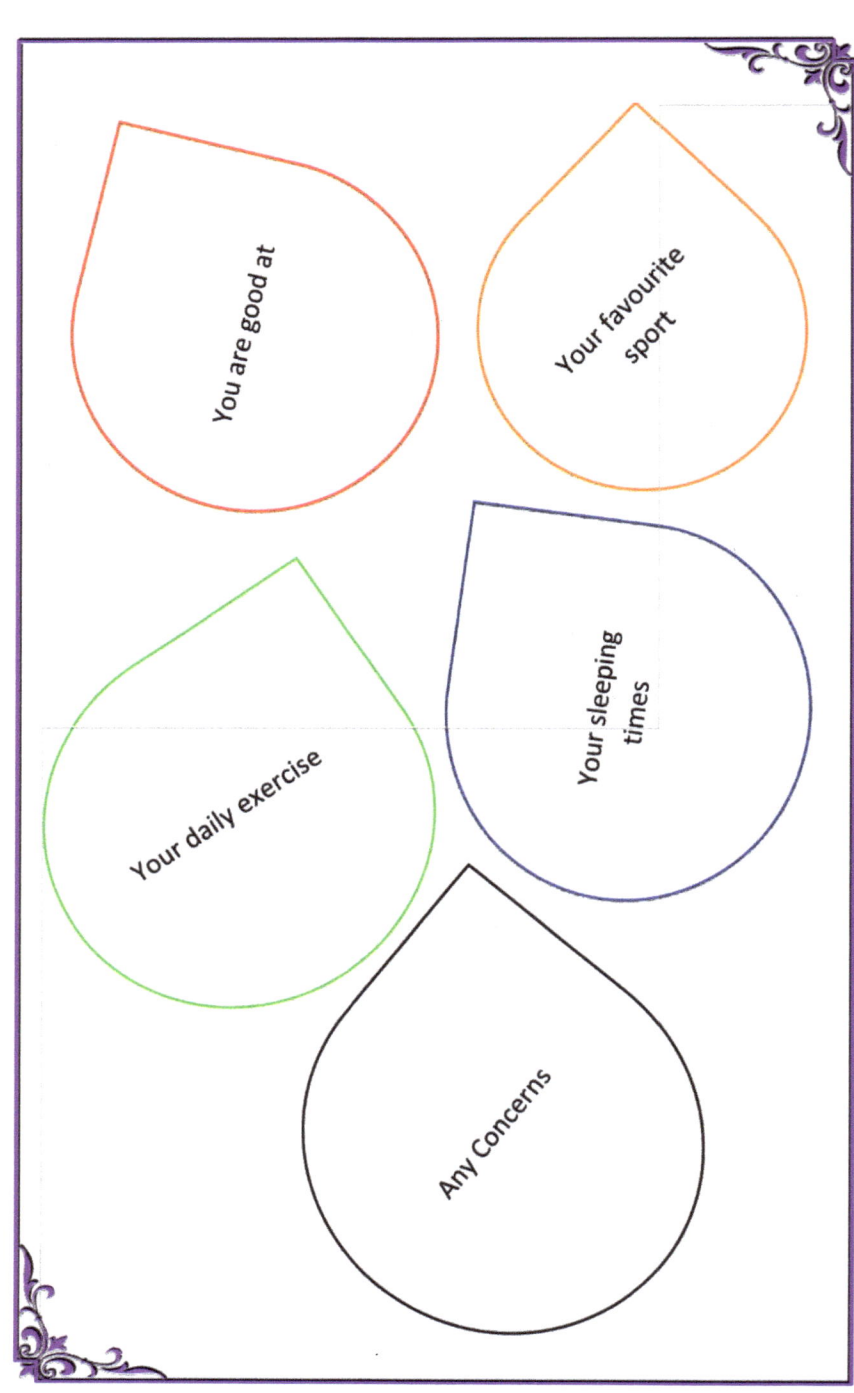

Hitches of the Journey

Contents	Page No.
Synopsis (what to expect)	7
Falls	14
Breathlessness	22
Joint Pain	26
Back Pain	31
Lack of Sleep	37
Fatigue	40
Forget fullness	45
Dementia prevention	51
Pressure Care	62
Incontinence Issues	65
Essential Tremors	68
Freezing in Parkinson's	74
Depression	77
Anxiety	80
Home exercise Programme	84

Ageing is a slow and continuous process of natural change that begins in late adulthood. During this age, many bodily functions start to decline gradually.

What to Expect

➢ Poor Balance – reduced muscle strength

➢ Slowed responses

➢ Poor vision

➢ Reduced hearing

➢ Changes in cognition

➢ Forgetfulness

➢ Urinary problems – incontinence issue

What to do

❖ For example, if you feel something that is not
> right with your body, you should investigate this with your doctor without delay.

❖ If you have any concerns about your medication
> and its side effects, continue taking your medication as usual and make an appointment with your doctor to discuss.

❖ Improve your bone health by eating a healthy
diet high in calcium and vitamin D. This means three servings of dairy products. Vitamin D comes in fish oils, fortified milk, cereals and from exposure to sunlight.

❖ Have your hearing and eyesight checked regularly.

❖ Know your limits as stress and tiredness can
make it more challenging to communicate. Take a rest or ask for help if you need to.

❖ When you are planning social events, make
sure you give yourself extra rest time beforehand.

❖ Always keep an appropriate identification, including your name, address and an emergency contact number. You could use an identity bracelet or necklace Pendant alarms to wear in case of an emergency if you are at risk of falls.

❖   Telephones with a set of large numbers or large
   auto-dial buttons with individual's photos or names are easy to use as you do not need to remember the number, just the person.

❖   A mobile phone has many advantages over landlines. You can keep it in your pocket. You can have a contact list, and when a person calls, their name and picture show on the display screen. On some mobiles, you can use voice activation for dialling numbers automatically.

❖   Sensors that monitor smoke, gas, flooding and
   intruders can reduce risks of accidents or damage occurring.

❖   You can use timers for heaters and electric fires

❖   Avoid using electric blankets, mainly if you are
   at risk of becoming incontinent during the night. If you want to use an electric blanket, use a timer to ensure it turns off.

Points to Remember

What to focus on

_____

_____

_____

_____

Mindful steps (important information related to you))

Not to Ignore

Nutrition

} A poor diet reduces energy levels and the ability to think clearly.

} Deficiency in nutrients can cause weakness or dizziness.

} Poor diet also impacts recovery time from illness or injury.

Osteoporosis is a result of general degenerative changes in bones and cartilages. In simple terms, it means bones are weaker, more fragile and are at higher risk from injury after a fall.

For some people, it also means pain in weight-bearing joints like the Knee and Ankle. Most of the general population gets relief after taking some non-steroidal anti-inflammatory over the counter medicine. But if the pain persists long term, do not ignore it and consult with your physician.

Cancer

Cancer can be defined as uncontrolled growth in a body without a definite known cause. It is treatable in some cases if detected early. It is essential to pay attention to all the possible warning signs of cancer like: -

1. A wound that is not healing or a lump that is unusual in shape, size, growth, or pattern is getting bigger.

2. A Lump or growth in the body especially applies to the breast for women and the testicles for men.

3. Unusual Discharge from any Body Opening

4. Any significant change in bowel or bladder habits

5. A Persistent Cough or Hoarseness.

6. Difficulty in Swallowing or Persistent Indigestion.

7. Any Change in a Wart or Mole.

Any mole that becomes more significant and bleeds or becomes an open sore should be considered suspicious.

Points to Muse

Any Early signs

_____

_____

_____

_____

Mindful steps (important information related to you)

Falls

Falls are a significant cause of accidental injury and death in the elderly. It is estimated that injury results from approximately 30% of falls, with at least 95% of hip fractures resulting from a fall. Falls are costly in terms of loss of function and quality of life at an individual level and care costs to the community. Roughly one-third of people over 60 years fall each year, with falls incidence increasing with age. People with a history of falls are more likely to fall again, with small cohorts who fall multiple times.

- Notably, the current knowledge base tells us that while men have higher reported rates of falls, women have higher fracture rates associated with falls.
- Falls are the leading cause of injuries in older adults
- Falls can be predicted and prevented

Personal risk Factors: -

- Fear of falling
- History of falls
- Increasing age

- Reduced hearing & vision
- Balance
- Urinary problems
- Medication
- Nutrition

Falls Prevention strategies: -

- It is essential to switch on dim light in the surrounding area before moving, especially during the night.
- Ensure furniture in the home is secure enough to support you should you need to lean on them if you lose your Balance.
- The flooring should be in good condition.
- Keep your living areas free from clutter.
- Remove loose mats and rugs.
- Ensure unobstructed access to light switches, window, curtains and electrical sockets.
- Ensure enough lighting for the day and night.
- Secure loose electrical wires.

- Tape a bright-coloured strip if the floor changes levels or if there is a slope.

Footwear and Indoor Mobility: -

- Wear comfortable firm fitting flat shoes with a broad heel and soles that grip.
- Wear shoes with a low heel. A broad low heel provides stability and distributes pressure better on foot.
- Ensure your shoe has a flexible, cushioned, non-slip sole. It will provide stability and shock absorption.
- Choose shoes with laces, buckles, elastic or Velcro.
- Never walk in socks only. They can cause you to slip quite easily.

Dressing and getting-in-out of the chair: -

* Do not sit on a chair that is too low.
* Get dressed and undressed while sitting.
* Sit up before you stand up from the bed.
* If you feel dizzy, wiggle your toes and wait for the dizziness to settle ultimately before standing

* The bed should be a proper height to stand up from.
* A firm mattress may provide more support for moving in bed and standing.

Getting up in the night: -

- Avoid getting up at night if possible.
- Minimise the distance you need to travel.
- Can you quickly turn on a light before you get up?
- Use night lights to illuminate the path.
- Sufficient time should be given for eyes to adjust to lighting.
- Ensure your glasses, footwear, and walking aid are bedside your bed.
- Take your time and do not change posture and position suddenly.

General safety in the bathroom: -

- Remove throw rugs.
- Wipe up spills immediately – do not walk on a wet floor.
- Remove clutter, e.g., plants, ornaments, floor shelving.

- Be cautious of detergent used to wash bathroom floor-avoid detergents which make floors slippery.

- Avoid using talcum powder on tiles.

- Use a non-slip mat.

- Be careful stepping in and out of the bath/shower. Install grab rails on the wall, if needed.

- Make sure you can easily reach soaps and sponges – Consider a soap dispenser/soap on a rope, long-handled sponge.

- Keep a towel close by so you can dry yourself before getting out.

- Use an assistive device like a shower chair and bath lift.

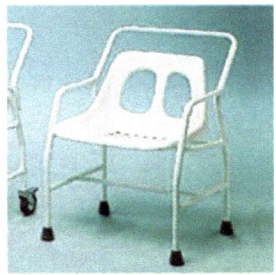 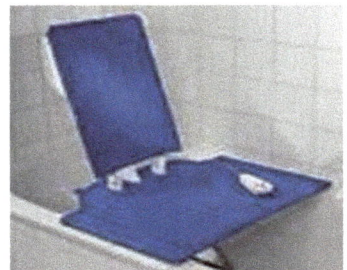

Safety in Kitchen: -

- Ideally, your fridge, cooker and sink should be in a triangle. Consider the position of other appliances in the kitchen, e.g., kettle, toaster, microwave.

- Arrange your kitchen so the most frequently used items are easy to reach and on the lower cabinet shelves.

- Ask someone to reach something up high for you. Never stand on a chair or overreach.

- Make sure you can open and close cupboards comfortably.

- Sit down when doing kitchen activities that take some time, e.g., peeling vegetables and washing up.

- Avoid carrying objects around the kitchen; use a kitchen trolley if possible.

- Ensure the mop and bucket is easy to access to clear up spills.

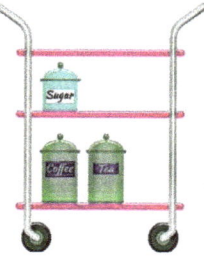

Points to focus

History of falls
_____

_____

_____

Mindful steps

Let's talk about the future

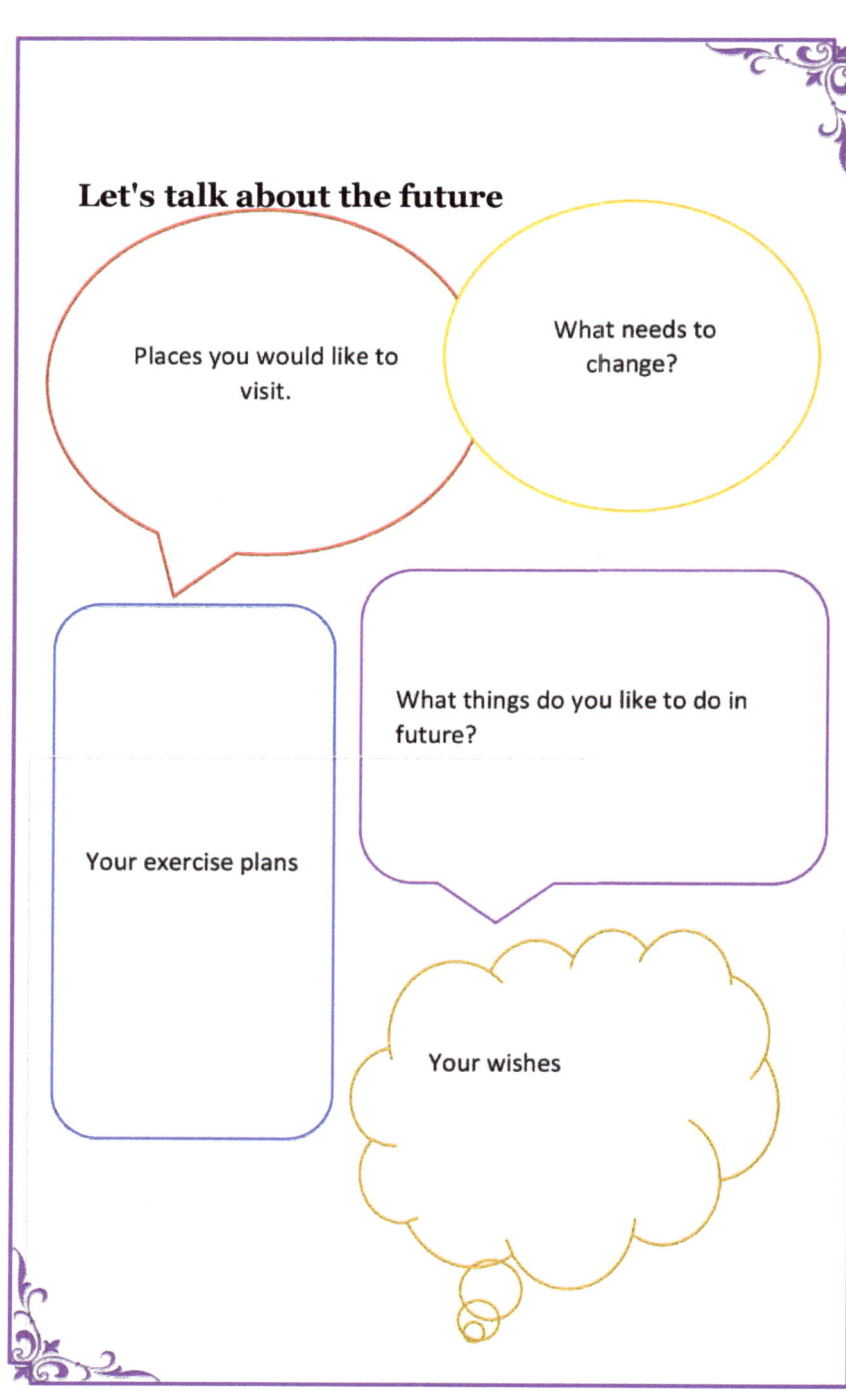

Breathlessness

Plan and Organise

- Plan: give yourself time to get ready instead of rushing and exacerbating your breathlessness.
- Review the set up for the task. Is there a better way you could do this?
- Plan, arrange and organise needed items before to decrease the energy required for the task.

Prioritise & adjust your Pace

- Look at all the stages of your personal care task and which parts are most important to you. Prioritise them in this way, e.g., you may choose to have someone assist you or structure as needed.
- Listen to your body

Delegate if possible

- Know your limits.
- Think about asking someone who can help. Try to delegate, if applicable, e.g., relative/ friend.

Adapt

- Think about choosing items of clothing that require less physical effort to put on and off, e.g., loose trousers, things with no buttons.

- Consider alternative footwear that does not have laces or buckles to be tied or use elastic laces where possible.

- Consider using some small aids to help with dressing, mainly to eliminate any bending and reaching, which may exacerbate your breathing difficulties (e.g., sock aid, shoehorn, Reacher).

Rest & Relax in between activities

- Take regular breaks throughout the task.
- Recover your breath before moving to the next task.
- Use relaxation exercises as applicable.

Visitors

Visitors can be enjoyable but tiring. Here are some tips to help you enjoy visits from friends and family.

* Limit the length of visits.

* It can help request visitors to come at times of the day when you have more energy.

* Have tea/coffee/mugs set out so that visitors can help themselves? Waiting on visitors is tiring, and most visitors would be happy to get themselves and you a cup of tea.

* Enlist the help of family to ask people to leave when you are becoming tired. It may be helpful to arrange a 'signal' to indicate when it is time for visitors to be asked to leave.

* Show peoples these suggestions when they come to visit.

Points to be aware of: -

Frequency of Breathlessness
_____

_____

_____

Mindful steps

Joint Pains

Arthritic joints cannot tolerate movement or any kind of stress like push, pull or twist. Taking time to think ahead and Plan may help you reduce your arthritis pain. These are some of the strategies that are advised by occupational therapists in managing your arthritic pains: -

1: Try to move each joint through its full range of motion (without pain) at least once a day.

The amount you can move each joint without rheumatoid arthritis pain may vary from day to day — take care not to overdo it. Keep movements slow and gentle — sudden jerking or bouncing can hurt your joints.

2: Try to understand the cause and factors responsible for pain.

Pain that lasts more than an hour or after an event may indicate that the activity was too stressful. Think of ways that you can modify the action. Remember that you are more likely to damage your joints when they are painful and swollen.

3: Always use the strongest joint or muscles available to carry out day to day tasks.

Be careful how you use your hands: -

a. Make sure not to push other fingers toward your little finger to protect smaller joints.

b. Avoid making a tight fist. Use tools with thick or specifically designed handles, which make them easier to hold.

c. Avoid hook grasp, i.e., do not items between your thumb and your fingers.

4: Use proper body mechanics

- When you are sitting, the proper height for a work surface is 2 inches below your bent elbow. Your forearms and upper legs should be well supported, resting level with the floor.

- For computer-related work, always use chairs with arms.

- When you are standing, your work surface's height should enable you to work comfortably without stooping.

- Use a highchair for sitting to decrease stress on your hips, knees as you get in/out of the chair.

- When lifting objects from the floor, stoop by bending your knees and hips.

- When carrying heavy objects, hold them as close to the body as possible.

- Maintain good posture in sitting, standing, or lying.

5: Do not keep your joints in the same position for a long duration.

For example, do not sit in the chair for more than half an hour without standing in between. Avoid long journeys in the car without taking breaks in between.

6: Maintain a balance between rest and activity throughout the day.

Do not rush in finishing a task at hand. Try to work things at your Pace. Rest before you become fatigued or sore—alternate light and moderate activities throughout the day. And take periodic stretch breaks. One step at a time. You must make changes in your habits slowly.

Let's talk about your friends with similar problems:

- Friends with similar problems
- What helps them to relieve pain
- What works for you in Pain
- Your pain medication name

Points to Remember

Frequency of Pain

_____

_____

_____

_____

Mindful steps

Back Pain

Pain is infinitely complex and has many dimensions.

Back Pain generally falls into three categories: -

Acute › Sub-acute › Stable

Acute: - Avoid unnecessary activities.

Sub-acute: - It is important to remember that even during the sub-acute stage, you must choose your activities carefully and choose new activities after consulting with your therapist.

Stable: - Do not take the absence of symptoms to mean that you can return to performing tasks in the same stressful manner as you did before your back pain occurred

Management strategies advised by Professionals -

- When in acute pain, bed rest is advisable.
- Do not sleep on your stomach.
- Sleep on a flat, firm mattress.
- Start some level of activity once the pain level subsides.

- A balance of rest and activity is vital to prevent further episodes.
- Avoid sitting in the acute stage but can sit for short periods, if necessary.
- When sitting, make sure that the lumbar curve is maintained. You can use a supportive roll or pillow if required.
- Avoid sitting in a low and soft chair/sofa. Always sit in a straight chair with a firm back.
- While sitting, make sure that your knees are higher than your hips.
- Do not sit in the same position for prolonged periods.
- Avoid sitting in swivel chairs and chairs on the roller.
- Avoid driving for long distances.
- Push the front seat of your car forward so that your knees will be higher than your hips. It will reduce the strain on the back and shoulder muscles.

- Avoid forward bending or stooping
- Lift with your legs, not with your back
- Fold your knees if you need to pick some items off the floor
- Do not stand in the same position for more extended periods
- Carefully judge the height of kerbs before stepping up or down
- Women should change to low heels frequently
- A hot bath or a warm shower will be helpful to decrease the pain
- Plan your movements ahead of time
- Do not carry a heavy basket or laundry
- Maintain a broad, stable base while standing and lifting
- Pivot your feet, do not twist your back.
- Keep your stomach muscles firm while raising and participating in daily activities

Rules for Lifting objects during day-to-day activities:

1. Plan your lifts and remove obstacles from your path
2. Test the weight of a load before attempting to lift it
3. Ask for assistance when necessary
4. Keep your back in a balanced position throughout the lift
5. Use your legs for lifting as much as possible
6. Always keep items close to the body when lifting or carrying.
7. When lifting, keep the load as close to your body as possible
8. Tighten your stomach muscles while lifting. Don't hold your breath.
9. Avoid twisting back. Pivot your feet instead of twisting your back if you need to turn while lifting
10. Replace quick/jerking movements with smooth ones and minimise reaching and bending

Let's talk about your other Pains: -

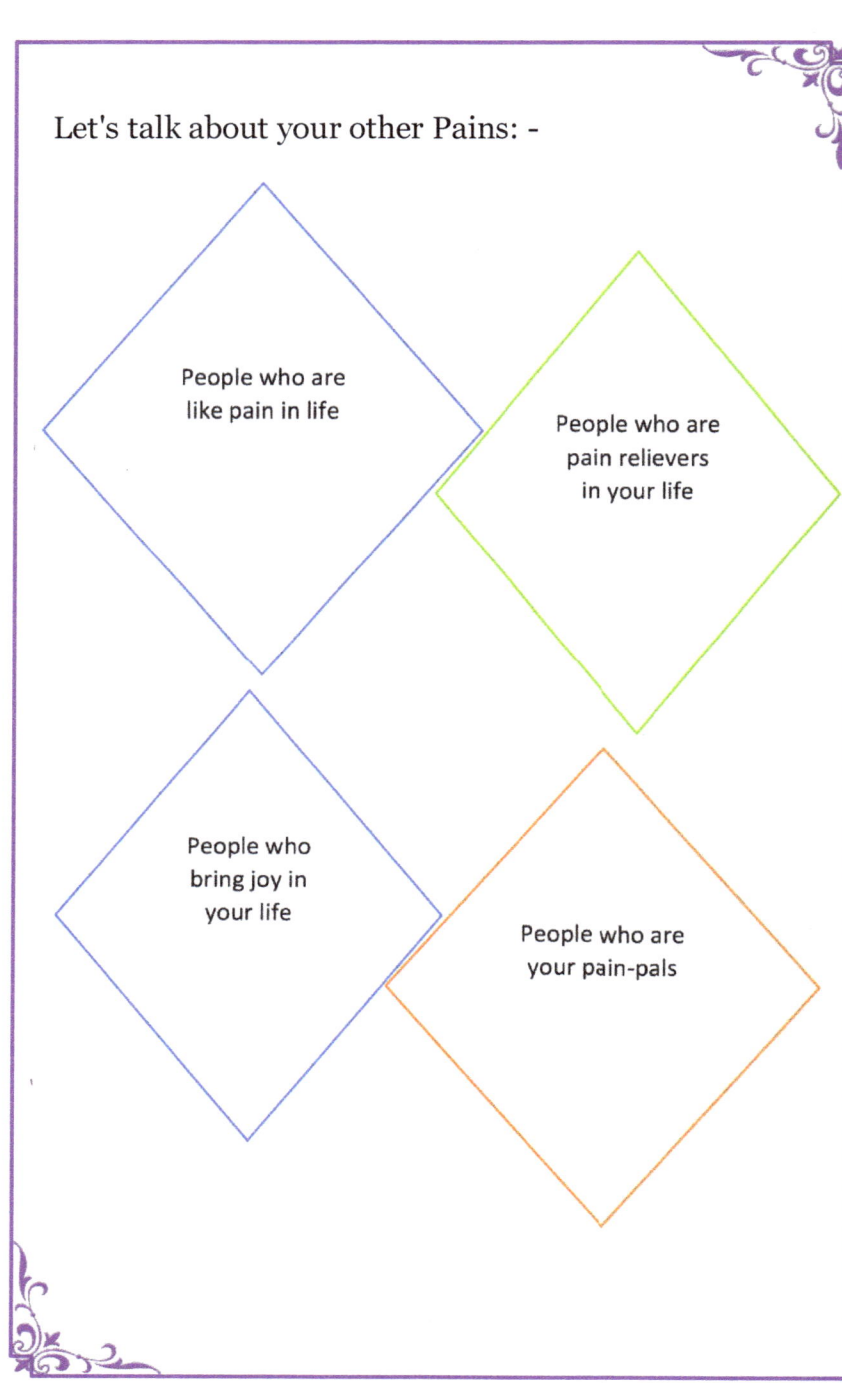

Points to Muse

Frequency of Back-Pain

_____

_____

_____

_____

Mindful steps

Lack of Sleep

What can I do: -

1. Keep a regular sleep routine – as much as possible, go to bed and get up at the same time each day.

2. Develop sleep rituals – this reminds your body that it is time for sleep. This might include a bath, relaxation techniques, deep breathing, or a cup of caffeine-free tea.

3. Keep bed for sleep – avoid using the bed for watching TV, reading, eating, working on a laptop or phone. Try to switch off media or gadgets an hour before bedtime.

4. Avoid Caffeine, nicotine, and alcohol (especially 4-6 hours before going to bed).

5. Environment – Make sure your bedroom is quiet, comfortable, and dark. A cooler room with enough blankets is best.

6. Eat well – keep a healthy and balanced diet. A light snack or warm milk before bed can help with getting to sleep.

7. Exercise – Regular exercise helps with sleep but avoid strenuous exercise 4 hours before bedtime.

8. Manage your worries –

- Talk with someone you trust

- Write your worries down in a notebook (if you wake up during the night with a thought or concern, write it in the diary and leave it there)

9. If you wake during the night:

- Use distraction techniques (e.g., count backwards by seven from 100 or think of people's names starting with every letter of the alphabet)

- Get up and try again (if you cannot sleep after 20 minutes, get up and do something boring, avoiding bright lights, until you feel sleepy, go to bed and try again).

- Avoid long naps during the daytime, if possible.

10. Drink less water before sleep but keep a water-bottle at arm's length.

11. Keep the mobile phone in silent mode if needed to stay nearby. Do not check your mobile if you wake up in the middle of the night.

Points to Remember

What wakes you up in the night?

_____

_____

_____

_____

Mindful steps

Fatigue

Fatigue refers to a mental and physical state of extreme tiredness and lack of energy. Most common complaints reported by people: -

* I do not know why I feel so tired
* I do not get anything done. I feel guilty
* Stairs seem like a hill
* I feel irritated with friends & family
* I do not feel about going out.
* It is time to think about your day and note down your symptoms.

Management of Fatigue: -

➢ Make a diary and write down everything you have done; from the moment you get up, you go to bed.

➢ Rate how tired you feel after each task (1-5).

➢ Prioritise your work, plan for the week.

➢ Do the task that you most want to do at the times of the day when you have the most energy.

- Develop a realistic daily schedule.
- Find time each day for something you enjoy.
- Spread tasks out over the week.
- Do a little bit each day rather than all at once.
- Split more significant tasks into sections. Select at a time throughout the day or week.
- Organise your work area so that everything you need is within easy reach. Sit when possible
- Alternate between heavy and light tasks and Ask for help with heavy tasks.
- Balance exercise and rest and plan frequent rest breaks.
- You may need to rest after eating.
- Avoid twisting, staying long in one position, bending, or stretching.
- Reduce pushing and lifting heavyweights.
- Eat a balanced diet.
- Make time for activities that relax you, and reduce stress.

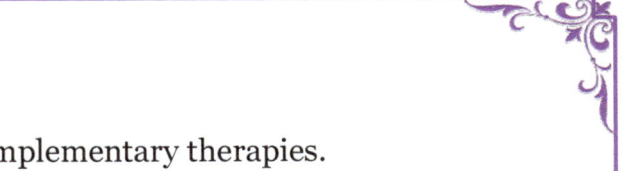

- Use Complementary therapies.

- Find someone who you can talk to about things that are concerning you.

- An Assistive device like a perching stool can be used to avoid long-standing in the kitchen.

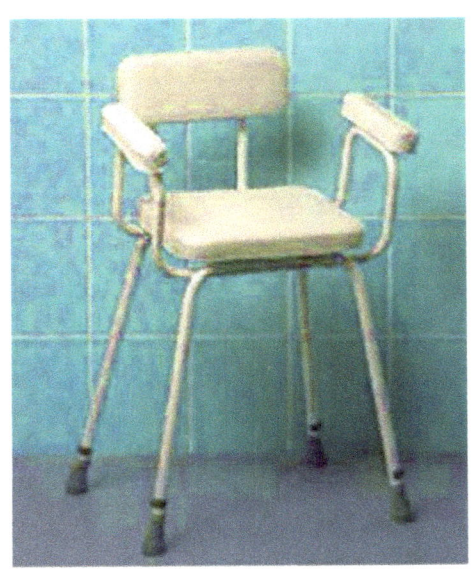

Rate how Tired you feel after each task (1-5)

*1*_____*2*_____*3*_____*4*_____*5*
Not at all   *slightly*   *Moderate*   *very*   *extremely*

Points to Remember

Prioritise you work

_____

_____

_____

_____

Mindful steps for managing fatigue

Forgetfulness

What can I do?

General strategies: -

- Maintain a Daily Routine.

- Keep things in the same place.

- Keep a Diary to note things and record appointments.

- Use yellow post-it stickers to remind you about what you have to do.

- Use a notice board to pin essential papers like appointments.

- Use pill dispensers or a blister pack to organise medications.

- Use labels for reminding.

- Make checklists of essential things to do before going out or before going to bed.

- Read newspapers or magazines daily to keep your brain active.

- Designate unique places for things you are likely to misplace, e.g. your keys, wallet.
- Pen or diary and find a way of marking this spot.
- Keep a list of where you keep things.
- Label the cupboards with what you keep in them.
- Keep keys on a pegboard.
- Be organised; give yourself time to locate items before you must do or go somewhere.

Meeting People: -

When you are in a situation that you can't remember someone's name, What Do You Do?

1. Do Not PANIC.

2. Go through possible names beginning with each letter in the alphabet.

3. Think of the situation where you first learnt the name and anything about the situation which may trigger or link their name.

4. If you still do not remember the name, do not be afraid to ask the person; you could say something like, 'I remember you very well, but your name has slipped my mind.'

5. You could tell your name as you shake hands with the person if it is your first time meeting them.

Seasonal Changes

In the summertime, very early in the mornings can be very bright. This can confuse. If people are not aware of the time, it can cause you to get up too early in the mornings, disturbing your sleep. Heavy curtains or blackout blinds will solve this problem.

Use Technology: -

- Calendar Clocks: which display the time, date, day of the week and month of the year. Position in a readily seen place, e.g., kitchen window or television on top of the fridge.

- Radio Alarm Clocks: can be set on the hour to get the time day and weather when you wake up. Set up an appropriate station once.

- Television: Turning on the television to a news station or breakfast show will usually have time and date and weather forecast to help orientate individuals.

Memory Tips for Maintaining Personal Hygiene

- Complete personal care tasks like showering at the best time of day for you. Whether it's in the morning or at night when you find yourself most alert and orientated.

- Be organised layout all the items you need for a bath or shower in sequence ask for assistance if required.

- Use simple step-by-step instructions and display them clearly for prompting and follow the same routine daily.

- You may find you lose interest in maintaining your hygiene because it is a difficult task. However, it is essential to maintain good personal hygiene to protect your skin and overall health and wellbeing.

- Develop a toileting pattern/routine to avoid incontinence.

- Wear clothing with elastic and Velcro waistbands so clothing can be easily put on & taken off.

- Wear/Buy clothes that are machine washable and need little ironing.

- For the ladies, front fastening bras are easier to manage, essential to wear a bra to avoid soreness, discomfort and skin irritation.

- Shoes with laces can be hard to manage. Using elastic laces may be of benefit or well-fitting slip-on shoes.

- Electric razors are more comfortable to use for shaving.

- Have a place to put dirty clothes to avoid mixing up the clean and dirty clothes.

- If you have difficulty telling if you are hot or cold several thin layers of clothing may be better than one thick coat.

Environmental Adaptations to Consider in the Bathroom

- Keep bathroom de-cluttered.

- Ensure there is good light, ventilation but that the room is warm.

- Put a sign on the door and keep the door open, so the toilet is easily identifiable.

- Put a sign as a reminder to use toilet paper and wash your hands. Make sure toilet paper and soap are in a place that is in clear view.

- To prevent falls, remove the toilet roll holder in case it is used for support. Consider installing a grab rail.

- Remove the lock from the door.

- Remove loose mats.

- Consider removing inward opening the door to the concertina door that can be opened from the outside.

- Remove all cleaning products for safety.

- Consider night light in hallways to guide the person to the toilet.

Dementia Prevention

What is Dementia?

Dementia indicates diseases affecting parts of the brain that are generally used for learning, memory & language, and day-to-day tasks. According to the World Health Organization (WHO), nearly 10 million new cases are registered every year and the estimated proportion of the population over age 60 and over.

Technically it is difficult with: -
- Reasoning,
- Judgement,
- Memory
- Usually associated with some other difficulties in Speaking or writing coherently (or understanding what is said or written), Recognising familiar surroundings; Planning and carrying out multi-step tasks

Preventing Dementia: -

Factors that are modifiable and can contribute to the prevention of Dementia are: -

1. Blood pressure--- Most of those who take antihypertensive medication take it for an extended period and sometimes forget to review it with their doctors. It has recently been revealed that some of those medications can be a contributing factor for iatrogenic (illness caused by medical treatment) Dementia. It is recommended that you talk to your doctor and see if they are happy with your medication or want to review them.

2. Diet-----Diet of a person is the most critical factor in deciding the long-term medical condition that a person can develop. Concerning Dementia, a Mediterranean-type diet is mainly recommended.

    It includes the following: -

- A large proportion of fruit & veg; Legumes; Cereals; Beans

- Oily fish (Rich in Omega3: -e.g. Mackerel, Tuna, Herring & Salmon)

- Dairy in moderation
- Nuts (Ensure you are not allergic to it)
- Poultry
- The minimal amount of Red Meat, Sugar & Saturated fats

Other essential practical elements that have been reported in preventing Dementia are:-

- Vitamins & Minerals : - Folic Acid, Vitamin B 6 & B12; Vitamin D; Magnesium, Vitamin C & E;
- Oils: - 1. Coconut; 2. Rapeseed oil, 3. Olive oil; 4. Polyunsaturated & fish related fats

3. Diabetes---Uncontrolled diabetes is also reported to be a significant contributor to Dementia. So it would be advisable to check your sugar levels regularly, even if you are on the borderline.

4. Alcohol – If you consume alcohol, you have to make sure that you take it in moderation. Heavy drinking is also a contributing factor in Dementia.

5. Habits: - The habits of a person are also a significant contributor to preventing or causing a long-term condition like Dementia, diabetes, stress, anxiety, or depression.

   Concerning Dementia, it recommended that you: -

- Keep a routine for your activities.

- Keep yourself active through your interest activities; Physical activity counteracts a major contributing factor (Apo E4) in the blood.

- Meet people to socialise and share a good laugh. Laughing is reported to be associated with boosting your immunity.

- Talk to people if you are finding some difficulty in your life.

- Keep a record of your good memories.

- Keep a scheduled time to sleep and relax.

- Watch the food you are eating and keep yourself hydrated.

- Make a habit of reading (e.g., Newspaper / Magazine /Book).

- Write down things that are important to you.

- Plan for the future and changing roles (Explore Assistive decision making and how to integrate into your will)

- Learning a new language or watching a movie in a different language.

6. Hormonal imbalance: - It is also reported to be a risk factor in rising cases of Dementia, especially in females. It would be advisable not to ignore symptoms and consult your doctor if needed.

7. Sleep --- Sleep helps you in recharging your body and mind. It would be great if you were mindful of your sleep timing and duration. Lack of sleep should not be ignored and needs to be discussed with your doctor. It is known as one of the significant contributing factors causing Dementia.

Some helpful strategies: -

- Always sleep around the same time.
- Keep bedroom temperature lower than your living room.
- Go to bed without any distractions like phones or books.
- Do not drink coffee or tea before going to bed.
- Try to keep a bottle of water near the bed to drink at nighttime.
- The bedroom should be in complete darkness during sleep.

8. Smoking-Avoid smoking if possible and avoid sitting in smokers' company as second-hand smoke & air pollution is one of the contributing risk factors in Dementia.

9. Socialisation ---As per research, people who are socially active & engaged are less likely to develop symptoms of Dementia.

10. Stress management: - Long term stress without intervention has the potential to contribute to developing Dementia. Some of the most commonly used strategies in stress management: -

- Yoga
- Meditation
- Mindfulness
- Walk

11. Physical fitness: Aerobic exercise three times a week - getting the heartbeat up a little bit is reported to help prevent Dementia.

12. Lifelong learning: It has been found in studies that those who keep their brains active are the least vulnerable group concerning Dementia. Hence you can choose what keeps your brain busy like: -

- Learning a new language
- Learning music

- Reading newspaper or Magazines
- Doing puzzles, Sudoku
- Playing cards and talking to your friends or family
- Watching News or TV and then discuss it with others.
- Write a paragraph every day if you can.
- Write a Journal every day, summarise the day, if you can.
- Develop a habit to write your tasks for the day.

Day	Tasks	Time
Monday		
Tuesday		
Wednesday		
Thursday		
Friday		
Saturday		
Sunday		

Let's talk about your life

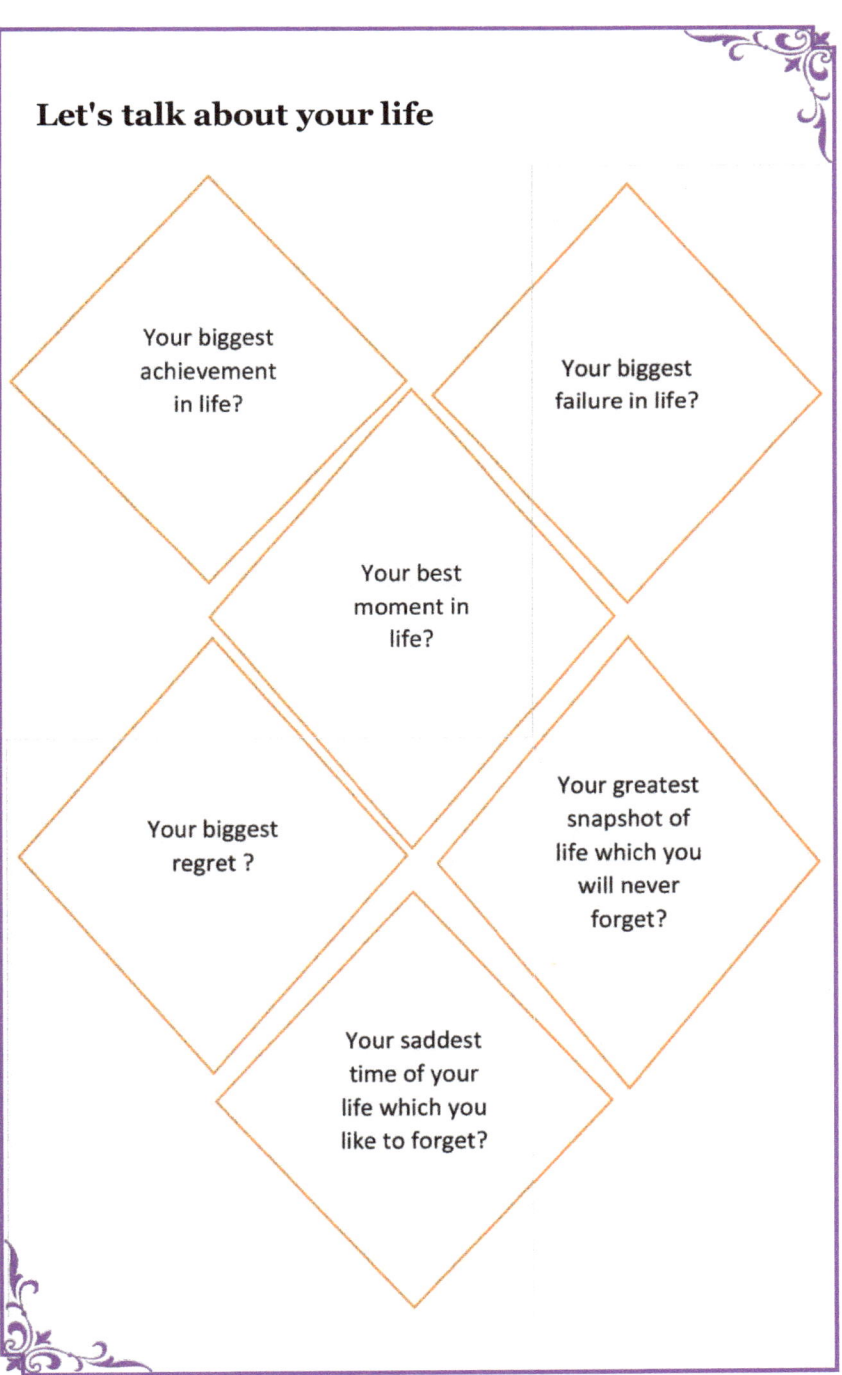

Points worth remembering

What do you forget mostly? (Make a list)

_____

_____

_____

_____

Mindful steps

what life style changes you do ?

Pressure Care

What is pressure care?

Pressure sores are common in people who are bedridden or immobile for a long time. They commonly occur in the areas where bones are close to the skin, like the sacrum, ankles, back, elbows, heels and hips.

These simple checks can keep pressure sores away:-

- Make sure to check your skin at least twice a day and keep it clean and dry.

- Change your position every two hours when in bed and every hour when sitting in a chair.

- Maintain good posture while sitting in a chair/ Wheelchair.

- Use cushions if developing redness on your bottom. Consult your nearest health care professionals if the redness does not fade with time or if the pressure area is getting worse.

- **Avoid:**

1. Avoid foam rings or doughnut-shaped pillows for sitting.

2. Avoid positions that allow you to slide or slump.

3. Avoid sliding with friction when transferring on surfaces.

4. Avoid vigorous massage, over a bony prominence.

5. Avoid smoking as it increases your risk for pressure sores.

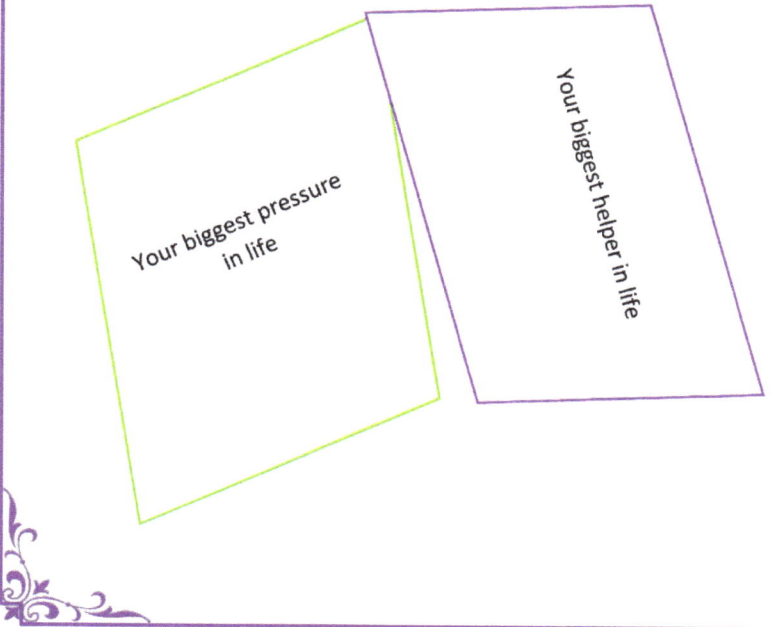

Points to CARE

Do you have any pressure areas & where?

_____

_____

_____

Mindful steps

Incontinence problems

Incontinence of the bladder or bowel is a common problem in Ageing. Pelvic floor muscle weakness is a common cause of these symptoms. The main symptoms are leaking urine with coughs, sneezes or exercise, leaking urine on the way to the toilet and wetting the bed when asleep.

What can I do: -

1. Drink smaller amounts of fluids at a time and cut-out beverages after a particular hour in the evening. Some foods can irritate your bladder, like soda, citrus fruits, and spicy dishes; Eliminating caffeinated drinks, which act as a diuretic, may help, too.

2. Eat whole grains and other high fibre foods to avoid constipation (which can add more pressure to the bladder) and go to the bathroom at more frequent intervals to encourage your bladder to empty.

3. Bladder retraining: - It involves keeping a diary of your bathroom visits and urinary leakage episodes. It also includes delaying bathroom Visits during an urge for a few minutes and overtime increase the length of the delay as possible.

4. Double voiding involves waiting for a few minutes after urinating and then trying to go again to empty your bladder more completely.

5. Kegel Exercises: -

    - Make sure your bladder is empty, then sit or lie down.

    - Tighten your pelvic floor muscles. Hold tight and count 3 to 5 seconds.

    - Relax the muscles and count 3 to 5 seconds.

    - Repeat 10 times, 3 times a day (morning, afternoon, and night).

Kegal exercise strengthens the pelvic floor & urinary sphincter muscles. If in doubt, consult your Physiotherapist for guidance.

6. Give yourself peace of mind by wearing discreet incontinence pads or undergarments to protect clothes and avoid embarrassment if you do have any leakage—this way, you won't have to alter your lifestyle and risk lowering your quality of life.

Points to remember

Have you assessed your symptoms?

_____

_____

_____

_____

Mindful steps

Essential Tremors

Essential tremor is a neurological disorder that causes involuntary and rhythmic shaking. It can affect any part of your body. It is often observed in hands when you do simple tasks, such as drinking from a glass or tying your shoelaces. The cause of essential tremor is primarily unknown. Here are some of the suggestions that will help you in managing them, if it bothers you:-

1. Try to learn using your tremor-free hand for as many activities as possible. Or use your tremor-free hand to steady your tremoring hand, and whenever possible, use both hands.

2. Avoid Caffeine and other over-the-counter medications and herbs containing ingredients that increase your heart rate and can increase tremor temporarily.

3. You can also try to hold your chin toward your chest to control head tremors.

4. Some people can control head tremors by turning their head to one side.

5. You can keep your elbows close to your body when performing tasks as a way to help control hand tremor.

6. You can adapt some activities, e.g., use bank cards instead of using or signing checks, if possible.

7. Always keep travel mugs with lids and request staff to pour tea when visiting café or restaurants.

8. Using sturdy thick plastic straws are also helpful while drinking.

9. Eating outside- Consider ordering finger foods or request meat be cut in the kitchen before being served.

10. Use weighted mugs or glasses for drinking.

11. Request staff not to fill cups/mugs

12. Use Dycem non-slip mats to stabilise your plates or saucer while eating.

13. Use electric shavers instead of traditional ones

14. Use voice-activated or speed dialling on mobile phones, if possible.

FUNCTIONAL STRATEGIES TO ASSIST IN CONTROLLING TREMORS

Typically, tremors are present in one or both arms, hands or legs.

A tremor in the arm/s:

- Apply gentle pressure through the wrist, hand, forearm, or elbow onto the arm of your chair or your thigh.
- Place your hand in your trouser pocket.
- Place your hand under your thigh.
- Manipulate coins in your pocket.
- Try doing a purposeful movement with your hand, such as combing your hair.
- Attempt one task at a time (e.g., focus on cutting up food and do not talk simultaneously).
- Be sure to take short rests during prolonged activities.
- Before and during functional activity, give the arm a good 'straightening out' stretch.

- When doing activities that require subtle movements, try supporting your wrist or forearm with the opposite hand.
- If the tremor persists, leave the activity until the tremor is more controlled at another time of the day.

A tremor in the leg:

- Sit and place feet flat on the floor.
- Press through the knees with your hand to push your heels flat.
- Move your feet in and out; stretch your ankle up and down a few times.
- Go for a walk.
- Rest.

When going to sleep:

- Gently press hands or feet into the mattress.
- Focus your conscious attention onto the affected limb and let it go 'loose'.
- Engage in relaxation techniques.

You may develop some of your own strategies to control and manage your tremors.

Let's talk about the most prominent tremors of your life

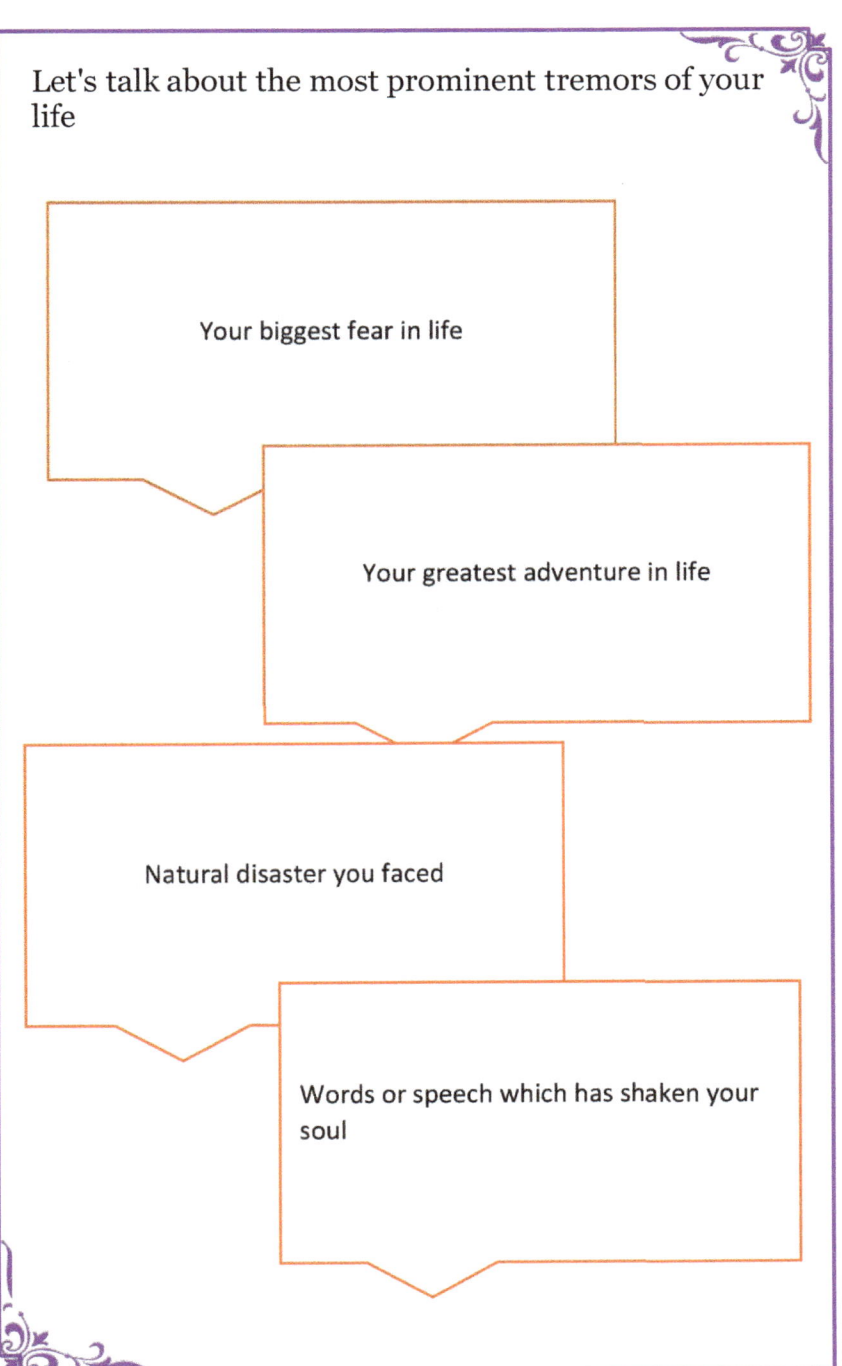

Points to be aware of

Things that help you to calm tremors
_____
_____
_____
_____

Mindful steps

Freezing in Parkinson's Disease

What is freezing?

- Feels like feet get 'glued to the ground' and cannot move forward again for several seconds or minutes.
- Feels like your feet are 'frozen or stuck, but that the top half of your body is still able to move.
- You may freeze when starting to walk or when you try to turn around. But freezing does not just affect walking.
- Some people may freeze during speaking, eating or during a repetitive movement like writing or brushing their teeth.
- Freezing often occurs in crowded or new places.

What to do when I freeze?

You could try the following method when you freeze

A. STOP

B. THINK

C. PLAN

D. DO

Let's talk about freezing points in life

Time when you felt numb or freeze

Points to Remember

How frequently do you freeze?

_____

_____

_____

_____

Mindful steps

Depression

Depression is a disabling illness. Those who suffer from it report that severe depression changes life completely. The symptoms of depression are: Feeling sadness/Anxiety, Lack of energy or motivation, disturbed sleep, negative thinking, unaccounted body aches and loss of interest in daily events.

The main symptoms of depression are:

1. A feeling of sadness and anxiety
2. The low energy level and feeling tired or fatigued
3. Sleep disturbances
4. Poor concentration
5. Loss of interest in hobbies, family or friends
6. Low self-esteem
7. Pain or body discomfort (Unexplainable reasons)
8. Loss of interest, suicidal thoughts

What can I do?

1. Lifestyle changes – Shower daily, change your clothes daily; make a routine for a walk & any exciting activity. Keeping your house clean. Make some new hobbies to keep yourself busy, e.g., Gardening.

2. Talk therapies- talk to your friends or neighbours. You can join a support group or activity group. Reach out to family, friends, or support groups to discuss issues.
3. Medication – Don't forget to take your medicines, recommended by doctors.
4. Does not sit idle; keep yourself busy, e.g., watch a movie, listen to music, go down memory lane by watching old pictures or videos.
5. Regular physical activity or Exercising is essential.
6. For a good sleep- shut down the media device an hour ago before bedtime, read a book or listen to calm music. Keep your room cool; you can use aromatic candles.
7. A balanced and nutritious diet – follow the recommended diet.
8. Avoid Alcohol -Alcohol is a depressant and should be avoided as much as possible.
9. Gratitude Journal- make a gratitude journal to say thanks to the people who help you in various life stages.
10. Having a pet is an excellent idea as pets require your care; they show love and affection and stay with you all the time. You can spend hours playing with them that distract you and break your negative thought process.

Points to Remember: What Can I do?

- Call or visit your friend
- Go outdoors
- Listen music or Radio
- Gardening or Cleaning
- Engage yourself in your favourite activity

Make a note when you are feeling down

_____

_____

_____

_____

_____

Anxiety

A certain level of anxiety is normal. It happens to everyone at times of danger or in worrying situations and can help in an emergency.

When we feel anxious, a chain of events happens in our bodies, which prepares us for action, also known as fight or flight response. There are three parts to the feeling of anxiety: physical, thoughts and actions.

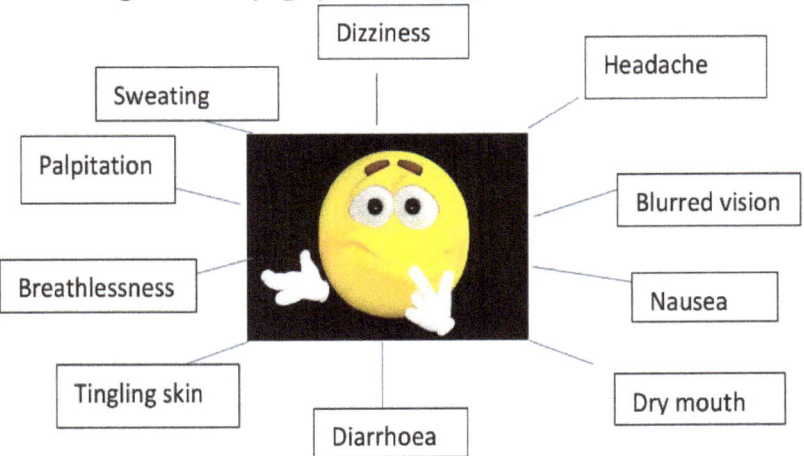

Anxiety involves a frequent, unpleasant feeling typically associated with uneasiness, apprehension, and worry. In some cases, people demonstrate physical symptoms like dizziness, dry mouth, sweating, tingling skin, tense muscles, blurred vision, heart palpitations, chest pain, shortness of breath and headaches.

What can I do?

Physical reaction, our thinking and our behaviour are all linked in an anxiety situation. How our body feels can lead us to think negative thoughts, leading us to avoid the same problem in the future. To manage anxiety, we need to recognise it and break the cycle as early as possible.

- Make a diary and write down what makes you feel anxious and how your body feels, and what you think at that time.
- Think positive- positive thoughts can help to relieve unwanted physical anxiety symptoms.
- Make positive phrases to say to yourself before, during and after the activity.
- Set small goals- when a task makes you feel anxious, it can help you see the job one step at a time.
- Distraction- when you are feeling anxious, distraction can take your attention away from negative thoughts. Select any distraction like – puzzles, crosswords, reading, knitting, sewing, listening to calm music or inspiring lessons, watch TV, talking to a friend or just go out shopping or coffee.

- Use relaxation techniques like breathing exercises, yoga, or guided meditation by visualising a peaceful and relaxing scene.
- Light physical exercise, such as a small stroll, helps in tackling symptoms of anxiety.
- Counselling can help people who experience anxiety frequently or Talking to someone like family or friends also helps.
- If the symptoms are not relieved, talk to your doctor

Explain your anxiety

1. What makes you feel anxious?
2. How does your body feel?
3. What you do, and what activities do you find challenging?
4. What are your thoughts, and are these thoughts reasonable?

Points to remember

Negative thoughts are like Velcro; unfasten them with Positive thoughts

My Positive thought
How can I Convert negative thought to positive
What activity can I do when I get anxious
What can I do to Avoid depressing conversation

Home Exercise Programme

Simple exercises for older adults at home

- Increase strength
- Improve flexibility
- Improve Ability to Carry out daily tasks
- Improve Balance
- Improve Mood
- Reduce stress/Anxiety

Exercise programme

- It includes 2 types of exercise:

Flexibility

- To stretch and loosen your muscles
- Increased joint mobility

Strengthening

- To improve your strength
- Limit muscle weakness
- Target arms and legs

How to complete?

- Repeat a few times during the day. You can even split up the exercises, completing some in the morning, afternoon, and evening.
- Several repetitions are required to maintain muscle strength and range of motion.
- The aim is to gradually increase duration. Make sure to check; how you feel during the exercises and adjust the level to suit you.
- The most important thing is to go at a comfortable pace for you. If any exercise is uncomfortable, stop doing it.

SAFETY ADVICE

- Avoid all jerky or sudden movements
- Avoid rapid twisting or turning of any part of your body.
- Listen to your body and take rests as needed
- Do not hold your breath
- Do not exercise if you are experiencing any of the following symptoms:

  o Dizziness

  o Shortness of breath

  o Fever

  o Chest pain
- If medically unwell, contact your doctor for further advice.

Let's get started

- You will need a sturdy and stable chair on an even surface.

- Watch your posture

*Sit up straight on a chair

* keep your feet flat on the floor

*Shoulders over your hips, make sure your spine isn't rounded into the back of the chair

*Breathe slowly and deeply

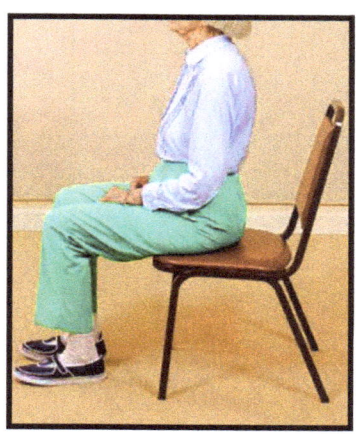

A. Flexibility Exercises/Warm Up

1. Neck Lateral Flexion

1. Sit straight and keep your neck and back straight
2. Start Tilting your neck right and left while keeping your shoulders relaxed.
3. Hold your neck on both sides for 5 seconds.
4. Repeat 3 times on each side.

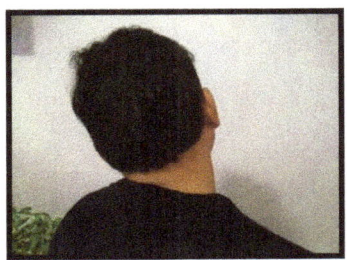 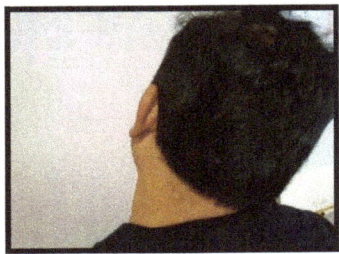

2. Scapular squeezes

1. Sit straight and Squeeze your shoulder blades together by bringing your shoulders down and back.

2. Hold for 5 seconds and relax. Repeat 3 times

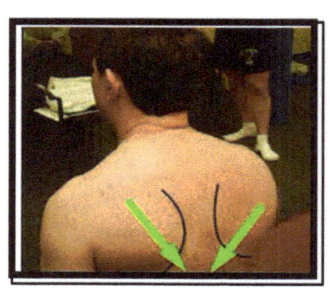

3. Shoulder shrugs

1. Roll your shoulders up and back.

2. Repeat 5 times.

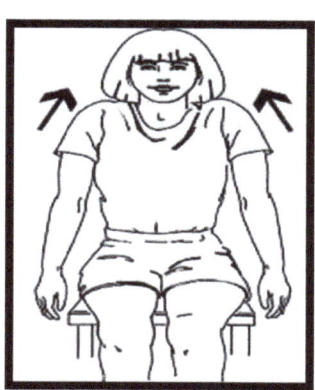

4. Overhead stretch

1. Sit tall   by keeping your back straight in a chair and interlock your fingers together.

2. Turn palms facing out and slowly lift arms up and down overhead

3. Repeat 3 times

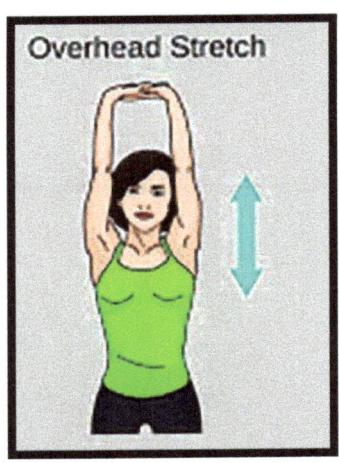

5. Trunk side flexion

1. Sitting tall in your chair.

2. Bring your right arm over your head and slowly reach the opposite wall. Try to remain in an upright position and not bend forward during the stretch.

3. Hold for 5 seconds, repeat 3 times on both sides.

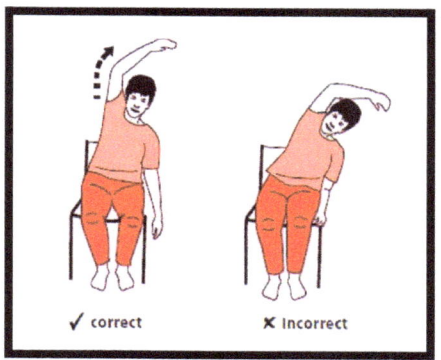

6. Hamstring Stretch

1. Sit in a chair, place one leg straight out in front of you with the heel on the floor.

2. Stretch your straight leg's toes and pointed up, knees flat and back straight.

3. Gently try to reach for toes and reach as far as you can without bending your knees.

4. Hold for at least 30 seconds. Repeat on the opposite leg.

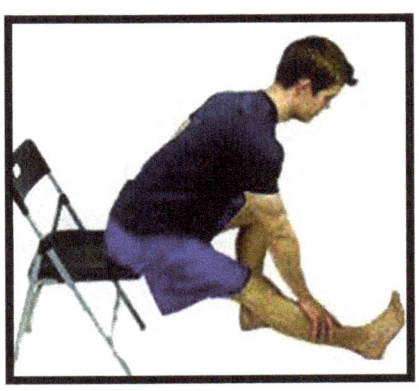

7. Knee Marching

- Sitting tall in the chair
- Hold the sides or arms of the chair
- It involves marching with your legs one by one. So you can start with right foot up and place it down. Maintain a rhythm that is comfortable for you.
- Continue for 30 to 60 seconds.

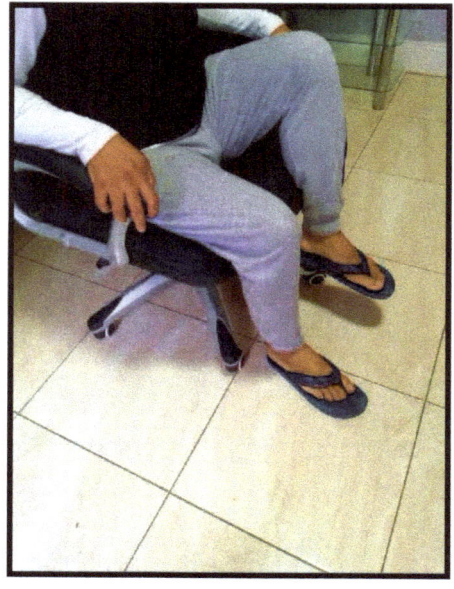

B. Leg Strengthening Exercises

1. Hip Flexion in sitting

1. Sitting tall and upright in a chair.

2. Lift your right thigh.

3. Hold for 5 seconds.

4. Repeat 10 times as able on both legs.

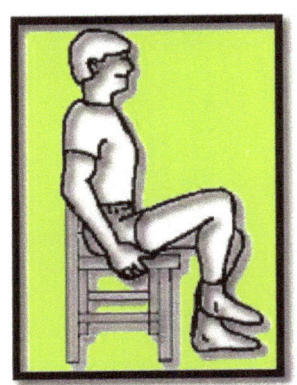

Progression:

Hold for 10 seconds   Repeat 20 times.

2. Knee extension in sitting

1. Sitting tall and upright in the chair.

2. Straighten your right knee.

3. Hold for 5 seconds.

4. Repeat 10 times as able on both legs.

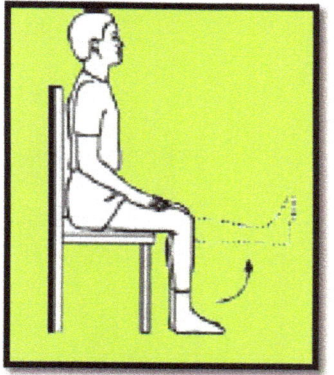

Progression:

Hold for 10 seconds   Repeat 20 times.

3. Sit to stand

1. Bring your bottom out to the edge of the chair

2. Always stand up by pushing up with your hands, keeping your head forward.

3. Stand up tall by straightening your back, tucking in your bottom and then straightening your knees

4. Sit down by bending your knees and reaching your hands back to the chair.

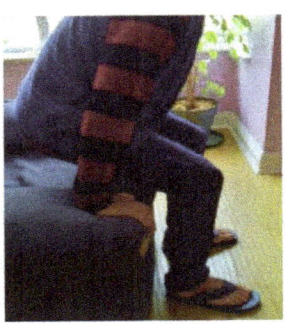 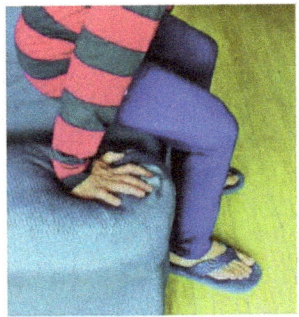

Progressions: Repeat another 10 times.

Only use 1 hand to help to stand or don't use any arm support to help you.

4. Toe taps/Heel raises in sitting

1. Sit tall and upright in a chair.

2. Tap your toes on both legs 20 times

3. Now lift your heels on both legs 20 times

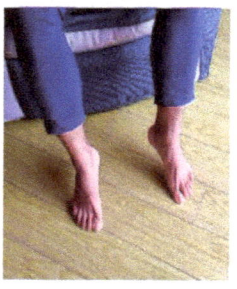 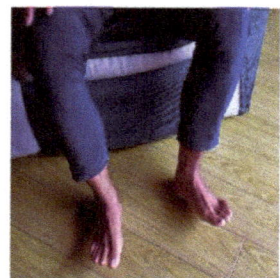

Progressions:

Increase the amount of repetitions you complete

Repeat the exercise again.

C. Arm Strengthening Exercises

1. Arm Elevations

1. Sitting tall in the chair.
2. Lift both your arms up towards the ceiling
3. Slowly lower back down.
4. Repeat 10 times

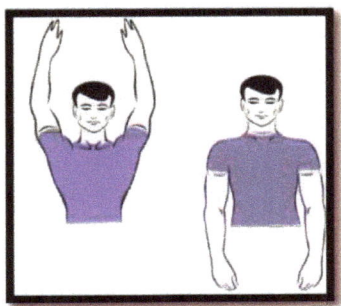

Progressions:

Increase the amount of repetitions to 20 times

Hold stick in your hands and lift overhead

Hold light weights (e.g. tins of beans, small water bottles)

2. Boxing position

1. Place your fists at shoulder level beneath your chin.

2. Smoothly reach your right arm straight out and slowly bring it back to starting position. Do up to 10 punches on each side

3. Repeat punching to the side and then straight up toward the ceiling.

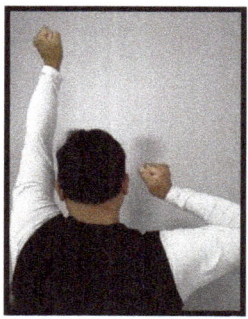 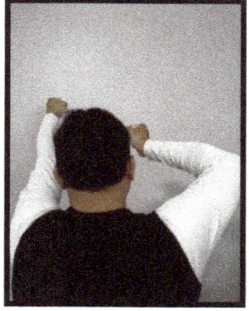 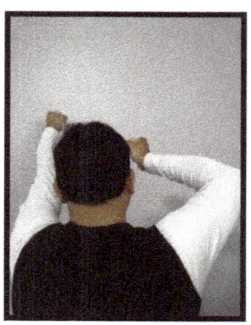

3. Elbow bends in sitting/standing

1. Sitting tall and upright in a chair

2. Bend both your elbows.

3. Repeat 10 times.

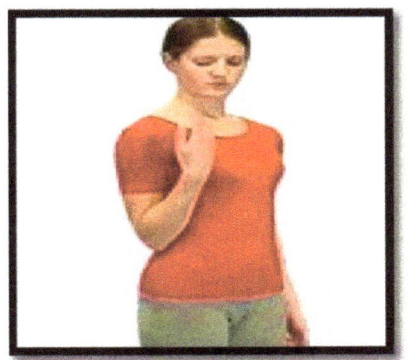

Progressions:

Increase the amount of repetitions to 20 times

Hold light weights (e.g. tins of beans, small water bottles)

Yoga

According to Indian philosophy, our life span is fixed and is measured not in minutes, days and months/years but in the total number of breaths. By doing yoga and retaining air in the lungs for a longer time, we reduce the total number of breaths during the day. This will help us to increase our longevity.

Other benefits of yoga are

- Relieves muscular tension.
- It improves lungs tidal volume & vital capacity.
- It improves oxygenation of the cardiovascular system & nervous system.
- It helps to reduce emotional stress, anxiety and depression.
- It helps in regulating high blood pressure & other heart problems.
- Amplifies the immune system by increasing the distribution of energy

- Refreshes the body and the mind.
- Calms and relaxes the mind.
- Improves concentration.
- Improves circulation. It makes the body function better.
- It helps to get rid of Headaches & Migraine.
- Promotes good sleep.
- Extremely good for the sinus.
- Suitable for the digestive system and liver functioning and diabetics.
- It helps to control anger & mood disorders.
- It is beneficial in arthritis, cervical spondylosis and backache.

Some yogic exercises can be done regularly:-

1. Sit tall in the chair, close your eyes and deep breathe in, expand your chest and slowly breathe out. Make hissing sound while breathing in and out.

2. 6-2-7 Rule:- Count number in your head. Breathe up to 6 counts, hold for 2 and exhale counting up to 7.

3. Breathing in through the nose and breathe out through the mouth.

4. Join both hands in Namaskar (Indian hello posture) mudra; fingertips and thumbs of both hands should touch each other. Keep this Pose in front of your chest. Breathe in, close your fingers and thumbs in and breathe out, extend your fingers and thumbs. Close your eyes and concentrate your breathing while opening and closing your fingers and thumbs

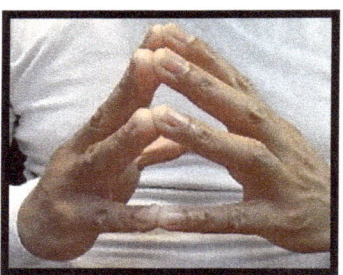

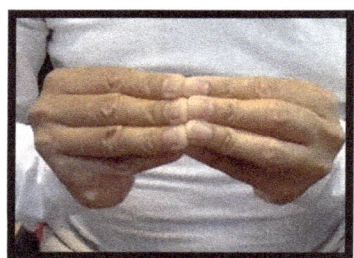

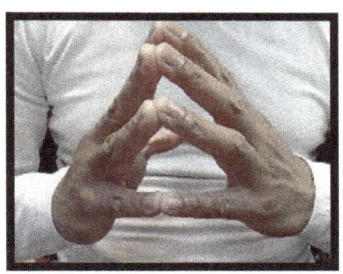

5. Anulom-vilom: - Close your right nostril with your thumb of your right hand (if left-handed, use left), inhale through the left nostril. Now close your left nostril with the index finger, open the right nostril and exhale. Directly inhale from the right nostril and exhale from the left. Keep continuing the same for 15 -20 minutes, 2-3 times in a day (Breathing from the desired nostril right or left-can be achieved by closing the other nostril)

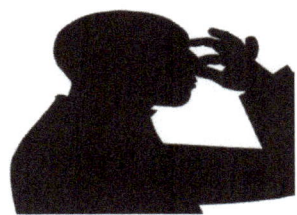

Long term medical conditions

Many older adults suffer from one-to-many long term medical conditions like arthritis, asthma, anxiety, acidity, peptic ulcer, chronic pain, heart conditions, diabetes, high blood pressure, irritable bowel syndrome, kidney problems, Parkinson's disease, stroke, hepatitis, depression, cancer etc. But everyone does not need to be going to get them.

The most common problems associated with long term conditions are Emotional difficulty, Pain, Fatigue, impaired physical ability and shortness of breath. Medical research has demonstrated long term long-term conditions can be managed by taking care of the following: -

1. Diet & Nutrition
2. Managing emotions

    (Grief/Anger/Anxiety/Frustration/Draining/ Loss of confidence)

3. Relaxation & Sleep
4. Fatigue Management
5. Pain management
6. Exercise

7. Weight Management

Some people take the challenge and become active self-managers and take care of their health and medical input. To actively manage long term conditions, we need two things: -

1. Active planning
- Plan something that you want to do
- It should be achievable
- Should be action specific
- We should be clear about – What? How much? When & How often
- Need the right level of confidence to accomplish a task

2. Problem-solving
- Identify the problem areas
- List ideas
- Select one & try it
- Assess the result
- Substitute another idea if needed
- Utilise resources available in the community

Active Planning:

List your ideas:-

1.

2.

3.

4.

5.

Select 2 ideas (mention why you have selected these two ideas)

1.

2.

Circle your confidence level (1-10)- (people with confidence level 7 and above are most likely to achieve their goals)

| 1 | 2 | 3 | 4 | 5 | 6 | 7 | 8 and above |

How and when am I going to do?

How often am I going to do?
Monday
Tuesday
Wednesday
Thursday
Friday
Saturday
Sunday

Assess result /idea (1-7):

Other resources (which you use for achieving your goal):

Success achieved :

Let's list your exercises Plan (2 times a day)

1.am
2.
3.
4.
5.
1.pm
2.
3.
4.
5.

Mindfulness

Mindfulness is the practice of paying attention to whatever is happening in the present moment and experiencing it without judgement.

Mindfulness is a practice that can help you to cope better with life's stresses. Studies have shown that mindfulness can help in dealing with stress, anxiety, and depression.

Many mindfulness techniques involve focusing on breathing and paying attention to develop a greater awareness that can help in the present moment. Practising mindfulness does not require a significant time commitment or special equipment. The goal of mindfulness is to become more in touch with life, your body and mind. If you are having distressing thoughts, do not forcefully deny them; instead, admit them and engage yourself to define them rationally.

Mindfulness is another way of paying more attention to what you do daily.

For example:

- ❖ Sounds and smells of having a shower.
- ❖ The sensation of your body while sitting down in a chair or putting cream on your hands and legs.
- ❖ Feeling your feet while walking at home.
- ❖ Noticing and appreciating trees, flowers and birds while walking.

Write your mindful activities of the day

Day	Mindful activity
Monday	
Tuesday	
Wednesday	
Thursday	
Friday	
Saturday	
Sunday	

The following few pages are for you to jot down information /ideas.

FOR MORE PUBLICATIONS

VISIT

www.newbeepublication.com

www.ingramcontent.com/pod-product-compliance
Lightning Source LLC
Chambersburg PA
CBHW061744290426
43661CB00127B/980